Multiple Myeloma's Natural Calcium Cure

Nomar Myeloma, Copyright 2019

Contents

Introduction:

This book is intended to give you a concise explanation of how and why Multiple Myeloma develops in the human body and how to combat the disease. Note that the author is not a Medical Doctor and can therefore prescribe no specific treatments or medications, however I can equip you with the knowledge to better understand your illness and to treat yourself with natural remedies and supplements! The information presented herein is strictly for informational purposes. I DO NOT BELIEVE MULTIPLE MYELOMA IS A CANCER, the symptoms of Multiple Myeloma have been incorrectly classified as Cancer and the disease is in fact a severe Calcium Deficiency in the body. When the deficiency goes untreated the body enters a state of chaos and cancer as it scrambles for the minerals it needs to survive, but when these minerals are supplied the body will restore itself naturally. I wish to remain anonymous as I do not want to be harassed and/or sued by groups such as medical institutions, cancer researchers, big-pharma and a litany of others who are in the business of making money off of cancer patients by "treating" their symptoms rather than offering them the real cure. Please excuse me for being cynical but I can't help but think that the cure has been known by others and perhaps even intentionally suppressed, the thought of which sickens me. I believe most of the Doctors, Nurses, and Researchers genuinely want to help, but at highest levels of certain organizations the true motive isn't to help patients and the efforts of most Doctors, Nurses and etc. can only go so far. This book is intended to be a concise and straight to the point summary so you can read it within a half hour and be on your way to a healthier you, I have tried to cut through the esoteric and get straight to the practical steps to recover from Myeloma. I strongly encourage you to do your own research and come to your own conclusions. Let's begin!

Credit to the Original Researcher:

Dr. George W. Carey laid out the work and explained how a Calcium Phosphate deficiency will impact the body back in 1894 in his work *The Biochemic System of Medicine*. I give Dr. Carey the credit for explaining this information and demonstrating the effects of a calcium deficiency in the body in a logical way. Don't dismiss the wisdom Carey offers simply because it's old material, newer doesn't always correlate to better! I believe this information was lost over the course of several generations. I simply stumbled across his work and realized that Multiple Myeloma is in fact a severe Calcium Deficiency as I had a close family member diagnosed with Multiple Myeloma and experiencing all the symptoms outlined by Carey. My close family member was initially diagnosed as Stage IV by one of the most prestigious hospitals in Boston, MA and is now in "Complete Response" aka fully cured but the Doctor's don't like to admit that so they prefer "complete response". My family members "m-spike" levels are at 0 and their bone marrow scans come back completely normal. The health of my loved one radically began to improve once he incorporated calcium supplements into his diet as part of his daily ritual. I will include some excerpts from Carey at the end of the book, they are a little confusing as they are written about 100 years ago, but his work is fascinating and well worth a read. His books are in public domain and some can be found for free online, I would recommend picking up a hard copy on Amazon of this timeless wisdom.

Symptoms of Myeloma or Multiple Myeloma

We are going to quickly summarize the symptoms of Multiple Myeloma only to compare them to those of a calcium deficiency shortly afterwards, as we will see a great deal of overlap.

Some symptoms of Multiple Myeloma (taken from American Cancer Society[i]) include:

- **Bone Pain and bone weakness**
- **Low Blood counts**
  - Anemia – too few red blood cells
  - Leukopenia- too few white blood cells
  - **Blood is produced in the bone!**
- **Nervous System Symptoms**
  - Sudden severe back pain
  - Numbness most often in legs
  - Muscle weakness most often in legs
- **Kidney Problems**
  - The bulk of these problems are caused by the kidneys having to filter out excess albumin from the body

Anecdotal Multiple Myeloma Symptoms

These symptoms are known to most people diagnosed with Multiple Myeloma anecdotally:

- Pain in back and Ribs
- Mental fogginess & grogginess
- Leg Cramps and muscle soreness comparable to lactic acid buildup after a workout
- Digestive Issues, hard to swallow, can't seem to digest foods
- Dental Cavities and Toothaches

Detection:

Multiple Myeloma is often detected or suspected when a blood or urine test reveals an abnormally high amount of protein in the blood/urine. The excess protein is caused by a lack of Calcium. Calcium and Albumin (aka protein) are the respective brick and mortar our bodies use to build bones. When the calcium isn't present there is an excess of Albumin and the Albumin has to go out as waste through the kidneys producing extra strain on the kidneys, more on this relationship later.

Calcium Deficiency Symptoms:

These symptoms are taken from D-cal's website [ii] and summarized below:

- Muscle Problems
- Fatigue
- Skin Symptoms
- Osteoporosis & Osteopenia
- Painful Premenstrual Symptoms
- Dental Problems
- Depression
- Difficulty Swallowing
- Chest Pains
- Chronic Itching

Clearly, there is some overlap between these symptoms and it makes one wonder whether the same root cause, a lack of calcium is responsible for Multiple Myeloma. Diseases are after all just a classification/name for a group of symptoms.

Original Excerpt from Dr. George W. Carey on Calcium Deficiency:

"*When the molecules of lime phosphate fall below the standard, a disturbance often occurs in the bone tissue and the decay of bone, known as caries of bone, commences. Phosphate of lime is the worker in albumin. It carries it to bone and uses it as cement in the making of bone.*

So-called Bright's disease (first discovered in a man named Bright) is simply an overflow of albumin via kidneys, due to a deficiency of phosphate of lime.[aka. When a Doctor detects protein in urine]

When the Goat salt is deficient in the gastric juice and bile, ferments arise from undigested foods; acids from the latter find their way to synovial fluids in the joints of legs or arms or ands, and often cause severe pains; but why the perfectly natural chemical operation should be called rheumatism passeth understanding.

Non-functional albumin, caused by a lack of lime phosphate, is the cause of eruptions, abscesses, consumption, catarrh and many so-called diseases.

But let us all remember that disease means not-at-

ease. And that the words do not mean an entity of any kind (ie: "cancer" that needs to be "fought"), shape, size, weight or quality, but an effect caused by some deficiency of blood material, and that only.

Phosphate of lime should never be taken in crude form It must be triturated to sixth X, according to the biochemic method, in milk sugar in order to be taken up by the mucous membrane absorbents, and thus carried into the circulation."

- **The Chemistry and Wonders of The Human Body, Dr. George W. Carey, 1921**

The Relationship

It is my belief that Multiple Myeloma is nothing more than a severe Calcium Deficiency that has gone on within the body for a long time. It is the starvation of calcium on a cellular level which throws the body into chaos as it begins to break down bone in order to get the calcium the blood, organs and muscles need in order to survive.

Calcium is a vital mineral for the proper function of the human body. One of the most important roles that calcium plays is building up our bones and teeth, supporting our immune system, helping with the process of digestion, and the proper function of our muscles throughout the

9

body. Needless to say, our blood has to constantly carry calcium throughout the body to where it is needed and if the bodies calcium supply falls below a certain level, symptoms begin to manifest.

Our bodies are designed with incredible wisdom built into the operating system in the sense that there are a number of "reserves" and storehouses for surplus materials that are needed for survival and our bodies instinctually know how to prioritize and manage these "reserves" for the sake of survival. For example, if one consumes more food than necessary, they accumulate fat reserves throughout their body, and in a period of scarcity or no food their body could survive off their own fat reserves provided that it had water, air and etc. We are not as independent as we may think and although the human body is incredibly efficient and wise when it comes to managing itself, we are ultimately dependent upon external resources for survival and replenishment; the most basic of these resources in order of Importance being: air, water, and food (vitamins & minerals). Without air/oxygen we are dead in a matter of minutes, without water we are dead in about a week and without food (vitamins & minerals) we are dead in about a month. We can however live for many years with a partial or incomplete supply of vitamins and minerals and symptoms and pains will begin to manifest, and will generally get worse if left untreated.

When one does not get enough Calcium in their diet, their body begins to take calcium from their bones. We could not expect our bones to grow dense and strong if we do not supply our body the material it needs to build bone. It would be like demanding a group of workers to build you a house when they haven't been supplied with any wood, nails or etc. Calcium is the main component of bone and without a steady supply of it our bones begin to deteriorate as our blood and other vital organs need the calcium to survive.

Within the body, the importance of one's blood cannot be underestimated as our blood is responsible for transporting the oxygen from the air to our organs and muscles, carrying the minerals and nutrients from our foods to the cells throughout the body and also acting as a general handyman and equalizer in the sense that the blood is everywhere and constantly supplying new material where needed and moving waste materials to be excreted. Ones blood is a living chemical equation that is constantly seeking equilibrium and which is primarily made up of water and minerals, the minerals each being used selectively and as needed to do a particular job within the body.

When the blood is lacking the proper minerals to do its work, its efficiency of operation begins to decline, and one begins to feel sluggish, tired and etc. When the blood lacks calcium from the diet it begins to leech calcium from the bone. The skeletal system serves as a reserve for calcium in the blood and the body will prioritize the maintenance of the blood over the maintenance of the skeletal system when its a mater of survival because without properly mineralized blood we will be dead within days or weeks but we can live a long time with a deteriorating skeletal structure (think gradual osteoporosis). Usually, under normal circumstances the body can "rob Peter to pay Paul" in the sense that calcium is taken from the bone/skeletal structure temporarily because it is needed elsewhere in the body and then later on the body will eventually replenish the bone/skeletal structure when an excess of calcium is available. However, when one's diet fails to supply the proper amount of calcium on a continued basis some serious symptoms begin to develop. **But my Doctor tested my blood calcium levels and they are fine, or even high, how can this be?**

Unfortunately, a blood calcium test has no way of determining whether the calcium in the blood is coming from the diet as it should in a healthy individual, or whether it is coming from the bones within the body; so it's fairly useless. The blood will maintain calcium levels by stealing calcium from the reserves in the bones as we mentioned previously when the diet fails to supply enough calcium to operate the body in its entirety. In fact often times blood tests reveal too much calcium for Multiple Myeloma patients. However, this is due to the fact that their bodies go into a state of emergency and begin breaking down bone rapidly to supply calcium to the blood but this cannot be done in a controlled fashion so more calcium ends up being released than the blood/albumin can use in a given time, so the body ends up needing to excrete some of it and the vicious cycle continues.

What about the M-Proteins in my blood? aren't these being caused by the "cancer"?

In order to understand the M-proteins we must first understand how the body builds bone and what it is made out of. Bone is composed of a number of materials but it is mostly composed of Calcium and Albumin. These are the respective brick and mortar that our bodies use to build healthy bone tissues. The albumin and calcium form a strong bond and the calcium serves as the brick and the albumin as the mortar in the sense that the albumin is soft and workable when its fresh in the blood but capable of hardening and becoming very solid similar to actual "mortar" a mason would use to build a brick structure which is soft and spreadable when wet but hardens into a concrete like mortar when dry. <u>Albumin is a type of protein</u> that our bodies utilize for a number of different functions.

Egg white is an example of an albuminous substance and anyone who has ever worked with egg white before knows that it is soft and plasma like at first but it changes into more of a solid when cooked, or left out to dry on cookware. The albumin in our blood is very similar in the sense that it binds to Calcium in the blood and then the albumin and calcium fit themselves into the bone to harden and support the skeletal structure where needed. When

14

the albumin is in its soft and plasma like state it can be used for a number of different roles within the body but once it becomes hardened into bone, it is no longer usable. Likewise, each calcium and albumin bond are unique in the sense that they are shaped to fit a particular area of bone and in the event that the blood needs to "steal" calcium from the bone it will need to separate the calcium from the albumin it is bound to, creating an abnormal waste protein in the blood which is merely the used up and hardened albumin/ portions of albumin that have been separated from the calcium in the blood. Therefore, it is my belief that the "M-Proteins" are simply pieces of hardened albumin that become present in the blood when ones diet fails to supply enough calcium from the body and the body then begins to leech calcium from the bones. See the following diagrams to get a visual of the process of healthy bone formation and also when the body steals or leeches calcium from the bone.

Calcium + Albumin Bone Formation:

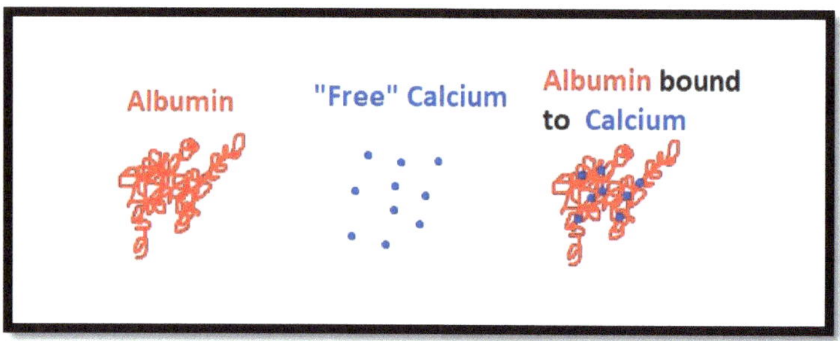

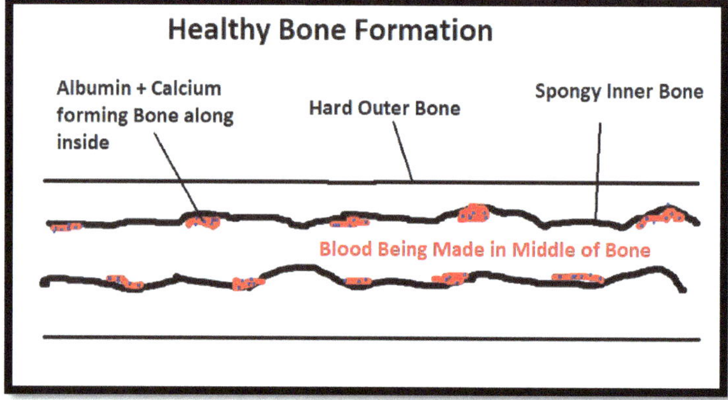

Bone Deterioration Visual:

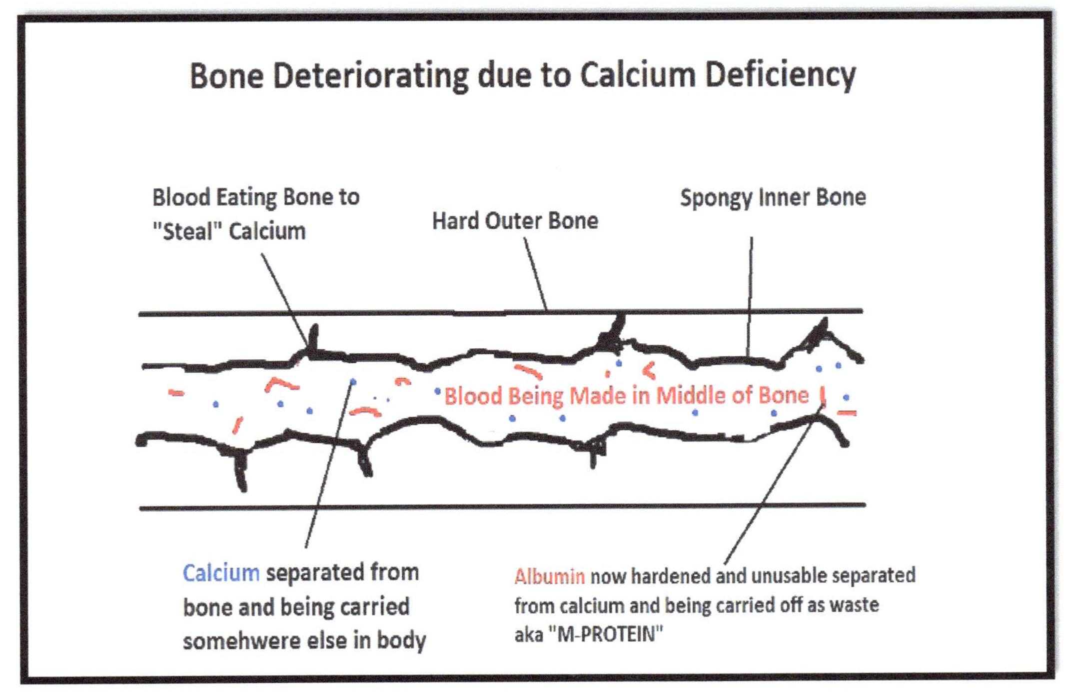

Summary:

I give Dr. George Washington Carey all of the credit for
elaborating and discovering the Calcium Cure for these
symptoms, I can merely take credit for re-searching
these brilliant old texts, translating his work into
layman's terms, and drawing the connection that
Multiple Myeloma seems to correlate extremely well
with the Calcium Deficiency Dr. Carey describes.

It was a really profound moment for me when I
came across his work at a time when a close family
member was diagnosed with Multiple Myeloma and I
happened to be very familiar with the symptoms at the
onset of the disease and could draw the correlation.
What made me even more convinced was the fact that
Dr. Carey suggests that a calcium deficiency is most likely
to occur in people born under the sign of Capricorn
(Birthday between Dec 21st-Feb 19th) which happens to
be true for the family member I know who that was
diagnosed with Multiple Myeloma. If you are skeptical of
astrology holding any merit in medicine, I would advise
you to do a bit of research and you just might be
surprised, perhaps the doctors in years gone by had
some wisdom that our modern doctors do not. After all
it was Hippocrates the "father of modern medicine"
(whom all Doctors even to this day take the Hippocratic
oath) who said "a physician without a knowledge of
astrology has no right to call himself a physician."

Carey, mentions that one experiences an outflow of albumin through the kidneys (through the urine), this is often the red flag that most doctors spot and correlate to multiple myeloma, high protein content in the urine. However, as he points out the albumin is simply leaving the body because the lack of available calcium for building and maintaining bone creates an excess of albumin in the body which ends up being disposed of.

Carey also touches upon the role of calcium in digestion in this excerpt and how a lack of calcium causes improper digestion which leads to acidic ferments building up in the body. I know that the person I know with Multiple Myeloma experienced this especially in the ribs and back (the areas closest to the stomach). In another section of Carey's work he elaborates on the vicious cycle of calcium deficiency wherein once it falls below a certain point it becomes very difficult for the body to assimilate the calcium from one's diet due to the fact that the digestive process requires calcium and therefore one needs to supplement with a form of calcium that can be directly absorbed by the blood.

Very important to note that Dr. Carey instructs us that Phosphate of Lime (Calcium Phosphate) should never be taken in crude form (ex: common Calcium Supplement) and only when it has been triturated (ground to a fine powder) to a certain degree. There have been studies done correlating calcium supplementation to heart attacks and coronary issues and I would never advise anyone to take a solid pill form of calcium that has a coarse molecular structure. The problem with coarse calcium is that is can clog the arteries because the molecules are too big for our blood/cells to move quickly so it takes a lot of time for them to move through our veins and arteries. Always opt for minerals that have the smallest possible molecular size so that our cells can utilize the minerals with ease and we can assimilate them with good efficiency. For instance if our cell's are the size of a marble and the molecular size of the calcium is the size of a golf ball, it's too big for our cells to utilize it. On the other hand, if our cells are the size of a marble and the molecular size of the calcium is the size of a grain of rice, it's small enough to be utilized by our cells. Yes, the body can break larger molecules down but its not an efficient process and its always best to start with a finer molecule and higher utilization.

I believe this is the way that minerals and nutrients are generally provided to us by mother nature (in a very small molecular size) in our whole foods and hence the calcium content in a serving of milk or spinach may only appear to be 10% of our daily recommended value(by weight), and a calcium pill could provide 100% of the daily recommended value, these "recommended values are only considering quantity and not the quality of the vitamins and minerals and I would argue that the calcium content in the spinach or milk although its less in regards to sheer weight will be a much more potent medicine due to the fact that it's in its natural state and small molecular size.

Therefore, I think that calcium rich foods are the ideal way to get your calcium, however foods grown in depleted soils are an issue today and the truth <u>is if you have a severe calcium deficiency you are going to want to supplement with something more powerful for at least several months until your symptoms begin to disappear</u>. Please note that I am not a doctor and cannot make any recommendations or prescriptions for your health, all I can do is share what my family member did to cure themselves of Multiple Myeloma.

I will say, that I personally use all of the supplements recommended in this book and not many Doctor's can say the same for the "chemotherapy" poisons they prescribe to their patients. I've never heard of anyone getting ill side effects from calcium supplements, especially in comparison to the horrible and often fatal chemotherapy side effects. I take no responsibility for anyone's health, you must think for yourself and act out of accordance with your own free will. Legal Disclaimer: Check with your doctor or health provider to make sure that these supplements will not interfere with any other medications or your health in any way before you consume them, consume at your own risk.

Great Quality Calcium Supplements:

Note that I am in no way affiliated with these products, I am only offering them to you as a friend on an informational basis. If I were affiliated with any particular product, I probably wouldn't be suggesting competitors alongside them. I sincerely believe that these some top sources of calcium and can help an individual overcome a calcium deficiency and restore natural balance in their body. #1 was the supplement that reversed the myeloma in my loved one and I have personally used all of the supplements listed below as a regular dietary supplement without any adverse reactions.

1) **Angstrom Minerals CalMag:**

It sells for around $33 online for a 32 oz bottle which should last about a month, maybe less if you are severely deficient. This is a potent blend of Calcium and Magnesium, of a fine cellular size that is highly utilized by the body. This is the exact formula that my loved one used to recover. **It is a very good idea to also supplement with Magnesium as Calcium and Magnesium work together in the body, and this is a great formula because it contains both minerals at the proper ratio.**

Dose used by my family member:1 Tablespoon mixed with a glass of water. Initially this was taken twice a day for several months and then reduced to once a day.

2) Sonne's Calphonite

This is a great liquid solution that is very affordable. I take it regularly and order it online through Swanson's Vitamins. This is the authors preferred choice as it is Calcium Phosphate and seems to be potent and pure and they get bonus points for using a real glass bottle.

Dose: When I consume this myself I mix about 2 tablespoons with a 8-12 oz glass of water. Again, I would take this twice a day if experiencing pain and symptoms and lessen to a maintenance dose of once per day when feeling better.

3) Hyland's #2 Calcium Phosphate & Bioplasma

Again order these online or your local grocery store may have them in the homeopathic medicine section. These are fine powdered tablets that dissolve in your mouth, I view these as more of a maintenance medicine that aren't quite as potent as the liquids in my humble opinion but still a great daily vitamin and great natural calcium supplement. The Bioplasma is a catch all blood mineral supplement with all the minerals required for healthy blood in the correct proportions that they would appear in natural/healthy blood.

If you are experiencing Bad Neuropathy I would strongly
suggest that you incorporate a good quality vitamin B12
supplement into your diet. I don't have any proof of this
but I suspect that some of the common treatments for
Myeloma rob the body of B12 and this is why
Neuropathy occurs.

What to Expect with Calcium Supplementation:

If you have been diagnosed with Multiple Myeloma, understand that you need to do a bit of catching up in regards to your bodies calcium levels and there is a finite rate at which your blood can rebuild bone. For instance, you cannot just gulp down several bottles of calcium supplements in one sitting and expect to be restored, as the body and more specifically the blood can only use so much calcium in a days' time.

There is a very real rate as to how much bone your blood can physically build in a day. Therefore, it is very important to stick with the supplementation, and your bones will gradually recover. I suspect that you will feel almost instant relief of some of your minor symptoms such as mental fogginess, and muscle cramps. If you are in tune with your body you may get an instinctual satisfaction when you consume a calcium supplement that just feels right and fulfilling and your body knows it is what you need. Within a few days your digestive power should come back to you and in a few months, you will be feeling like yourself again! Once you begin calcium supplementation you will halt the deterioration of your symptoms an begin the process of recovery.

I would also recommend taking a magnesium supplement too if you opt for taking something other than *Angstrom CalMag*, ideally the Magnesium would be in liquid form but a capsule or tablet will be better than nothing. You will need more Calcium initially and I would strongly recommend supplementing with a liquid calcium such as *CalMag* or *Sonne's Calphonite*, and then as you begin to feel better you can reduce to a maintenance dosage or simply just be mindful of your diet and ensure you get plenty of natural Calcium through your diet.

Don't dismiss this simple cure because it isn't a brand new technology or exciting medical breakthrough, the wiser we get we realize that many things have already been discovered in the past and the information gets lost or intentionally buried, hence the need for re-searching. Also don't be discouraged by the simplicity of this cure, in most instances unless we have been subjected to something extremely toxic (ex: radiation, agent orange, etc) that damages our body, when one becomes sick it is usually because one is lacking a vital mineral or nutrient in a sufficient quantity. If we are hungry, food is the solution! Don't assume that because we are more civilized and "high-tech" today that our Doctors are more educated and know everything. While surgical techniques and life-saving devices are certainly more advanced, that doesn't mean that our overall medical wisdom is much better as most doctors fail to understand the importance of quality nutrition and essentially skim over the importance of the basic vitamins and minerals because they are working under the false assumption that because we live in a first world country all of our nutritional needs are being met. However, most of us are fairly routine in our diets and we eat the same handful of meals over and over and we aren't truly supplying all the vitamins and minerals that the body needs to thrive.

Natural Sources of Calcium:

- **Milk**
  - Your Mother was right when she told you to drink your milk for strong bones!
- **Cheese**
  - Several Myeloma patients reported a craving for cheese, this is their bodies instinctual understanding that they need calcium
- **Bones**!
  - Use chicken and beef bones to create a homemade bone-broth souper-food
    - These are truly powerful and restorative as the calcium and gelatin from the bones really replenish the body, see Chicken Noodle Soup Recipe included at back of book!
- **Greens**
  - Broccoli, Kale, collards, Romaine lettuce, Spinach
- **Oatmeal** (One of the best things we can eat,Opt for old fashioned or Steel cut and don't overcook it (aka Keep GI low) and don't load it up with sugar!)
  - I enjoy my oatmeal with a dash of sea salt fresh from the grinder
- **Egg Yolks** (Also great for Vitamin D)
  - I eat about a dozen eggs a week, and my cholesterol levels are great, it is complete BS that eating high cholesterol foods lead to "high cholesterol." Cholesterol is a vital nutrient your body needs!

Dietary Advice:

Get your life in order and prioritize your health! Forget about the new fad-diets, if you want to learn how to truly eat to live, I would strongly recommend you go out and get a copy of Sally Fallon's book *Nourishing Traditions.* Eat foods that are fresh and rich with the intangible vital life force. Add meats to your diet slowly if you are recovering from Calcium Deficiency, as meats will require a great deal of digestive strength to digest properly. Start with softer proteins such as Eggs and Fish and work your way back up to meats. **If your blood tests show Anemia, you need to eat more red meat or take an iron supplement. There's no other way to restore an Anemic condition, other than consuming the iron needed to effectively transport oxygen in the blood.** When we lack iron we force our heart and bodies to work extra hard because we need to move more blood to supply the same amount of oxygen because the blood becomes less efficient. This often causes one to have a fever because they are pumping more blood than usual.

Anemia aside, Americans generally eat way too much meat. As someone who has tried vegetarianism for over a year I will say that we truly don't need meat to survive, however I believe animal meats and fats are a highly efficient source of nutrition and can help us stay in optimal shape.

We are animals after all and we are dependent on external chemicals such as air, water, and food to survive and thrive. The most nourishing of Animal foods are organ meats, particularly the Liver. When a predator such as a lion or wolf kills an animal in the wild, the first thing they eat is the liver. The liver is packed with nutrients, Vitamin A and minerals; it is one of the most nutritionally dense foods available; and it is also one of the cheapest foods available! Pick up some beef liver at your local supermarket, bust out the skillet, caramelize some onions and sear up some nice liver. It may not be the tastiest thing but <u>you MUST realize that good taste is not correlated to good health, in fact the opposite is generally true or rather bland and simple taste is usually the best for us</u>. If it comes in a package and is ready to eat, it is ready for the trash bin; if it is fresh and takes a bit of time and TLC to prepare, it is fit for building your temple.

Eat Simple:
Don't mix too many different types of food in your stomach at once. This taxes your digestive system because it can't do a good job of breaking the foods down. Keep your meals simple with one to two things being eaten at a particular time/ sitting. I am not saying have the same things over and over, this is a big no-no and a key contributor to mineral deficiencies variety in the diet supplies the body with a broad array of vitamins and minerals and is great for your health, just don't have too much variety with each meal.

Fast:
Fasting is extremely beneficial and helps our bodies to heal. Make sure you provide your body with the key nutrients it needs, but give your body time to recover. We must realize that every time we eat, we are using up some of our vital energy to digest foods. When we take a break from eating, we allow our vital energy to work on repairing and rebuilding the body. Don't take fasting to the extreme, like most things that yield optimal health it is a balancing act and moderation

is best. Try eating two meals a day instead of three, you begin with a regular breakfast (don't overcompensate by eating a massive breakfast), skip lunch, and then have a normal dinner. You will soon see why it's called "fasting" as you will have more energy than ever!

Sunshine:

One of the crazy and illogical fears of today is a fear of the sun. Yes, too much of anything good can be a bad thing, but the Sun is the source of all life on Earth! We feel so much better and our bodies become invigorated when we get a little sunshine in our day. Have you ever seen a plant thrive without the sun? Certain processes in our bodies rely on the Sun in a similar fashion. Vitamin D is a key component in building bone and restoring a calcium deficiency and unfortunately there is no man-made match for the Sunshine mother nature provides us. It is a good idea to spend some time outside and soak up some sun. I personally, never wear sun screen and instead opt to throw on a sweatshirt or move under the umbrella if I feel the sun is getting too hot. Try and soak up around 20-30 minutes of Sunshine a day. I also notice that the symptoms of Myeloma tend to be the worst during the winter months and I think this is part of the reason, we aren't getting enough Vitamin D. If you are wealthy and are struggling with the symptoms of Myeloma it would be wise to spend your winters somewhere like Florida where you can still enjoy the Sun. Use your head, if you have had skin cancer in the past, limit your sunshine and take a Vitamin D Gel Capsule as an alternative. If you have sensitive moles or etc I would consider getting a Zinc Based sunscreen stick to cover small spots such as moles, and other areas prone to burning such as your nose and etc.

Hydrate Properly:

Drink plenty of water, and drink only water, milk and simple juices. You don't need to drink a gallon or more a day as some "new studies" suggest, just don't allow yourself to go thirsty and keep plenty of fresh water on hand. DO NOT DRINK TAP WATER, buy clean spring water or drink distilled water, tap water is loaded with nasty chemicals such as Fluoride and Chlorine. My favorite is Acqua Panna as it comes in the glass bottle. Ditch the alcohol, soda and sugary drinks. Keep the coffee and caffeine to a minimum, you don't need it and when we rely on stimulants to boost our energy we do so at the expense of our inner energy and will power.

Keep Sugar and Carbs in Check:

Our bodies actually do need sugar to thrive but not nearly as much as the Average American consumes. Completely avoid Soda and liquid sugary cocktails as these are the worst on our bodies. The only acceptable sugar is really fruits and vegetables in their natural state. Fresh apples, bananas, carrots, beets and etc. will provide you with the best sources of sugar for your body. Keep the carbs to a minimum and focus on carbs that digest slowly and have a low GI rating. Study up on the Glycemic Index or GI of the foods you eat and replace high GI foods with low GI alternatives. Stay away from Bread! Bread is one of the highest GI foods we can eat and definitely not good for one's blood sugar and daily sugar intake. You need to prioritize your health over taste. Eat to live don't live to eat!

Consider a Detox:

I would certainly incorporate a detox into my healing regiment, if your intestines and gut are lined with junk food and decaying food, it won't be good for your body. This is particularly important for Myeloma patients because the calcium deficiency hinders their digestive power so foods will go largely undigested and will end up turning toxic inside your intestines. Imagine what would happen if you kept a pile of ground up meat inside a bag that was heated to about 98 degrees for several days, the rot and smell would be horrible. This is exactly what is happening inside our bodies when we fail to properly assimilate foods. Junk foods and residues will gradually build up in our intestines and this will create a vicious cycle where our digestive tract becomes less effective because there is less surface area of the intestines exposed to the food and therefore we get less nutrients out of our food.

To cleanse your intestinal tract I would recommend a an **Oxygen based intestinal cleanser such as Mag 07** which is available online at a number of major retailers. Use this for several days and eat light during those days and eat hard starchy foods such as apples, raw carrots, corn and etc. that will move through your intestines and assist with the cleanse. You will experience diarrhea with this product, but that is how it works and I never find it to be a painful or uncontrollable type of diarrhea. It would be a good idea to consume some fresh fruit and vegetable juices that are rich in alkaline salts and cleansing nutrients. My personal favorite juice is made with ginger root, beets, apples, carrots and lime. I feel fantastic when I make this and I like to enjoy it several times a week. You will need to buy a good Juicer if you don't already have one, *Breville* makes good juicers that are great for your in-home usage. These juices when properly made don't have any actual food that needs to be broken down by our bodies but rather they contain the vital essence and nutrients of a fruit/vegetable suspended in water, therefore it takes very little effort for our bodies to digest these juices and your digestive system remains un-taxed during your cleanse.

Another great and cheap detox is to use **bentonite clay,** you simply mix it with some water and have it occasionally. My favorite brand is **Sonne's #7** Detoxification. The bentonite clay moves through your intestinal tract and acts as a magnet for heavy metals and contaminants. You can also add this to a fresh juice but I prefer to keep them separate. I would recommend using this as a regular maintenance type cleanse several times a week. After the initial several day cleanse.

If you really want to get down to business and ensure your intestines are clean, you can look into a colonic irrigation which is essentially an enema which continually flushes and refills your intestinal tract with clean water. You will need to go to a local holistic medical office or etc to find one of these near you. I honestly have never tried it but I believe it was Andrew Carnegie who swore that they kept him feeling invigorated and mentally alert.

Exercise:

If you are experiencing severe pain in your back, ribs, legs and etc., exercise is simply not going to be an option. However, the simple act of circulating the blood throughout our bodies can work wonders for our health and dramatically speed up one's recovery. As you begin to recover, and feel your bones are ready for exercise begin to build up gradually with a nice walk/powerwalk around your neighborhood just enough to get the blood moving. Calisthenics such as stretching, jumping jacks, and burpees work wonders for moving blood throughout our bodies and I would highly recommend you incorporate these into your daily routine once you are feeling stronger.

Practice deep breathing and yoga to help still your mind and purify your blood. A particular yoga technique called breath of fire is a strong way of purifying and strengthening your blood by flooding it with oxygen temporarily. Search YouTube for instructions on this technique. Find something you like to do to keep your body moving, and your blood pumping, we need to use it or lose it!

Sexual Advice:

Less Sex = More Strength and Energy

There is a higher concentration of calcium in semen than there is in the blood! Not only is the loss of calcium going to be important, but sex, masturbation, and ejaculation for the sake of pleasure deprives men and women of their most precious life force. The wise men and women of days begone knew of the power of harnessing ones sexual energy and transmuting it into projects, dreams and tasks of a higher nature. When one is in a depleted or seriously ill state they cannot afford to "sow their seed to the wind" as it will drain them of their vital force which will be crucial to their recovery.

Every ejaculation has the life force inherent within it to create another human being! I believe this is the only reason why the medication Revlemid which is often prescribed to Multiple Myeloma Patients has had some benefit. I believe it has nothing to do with the medication but rather the fact that men are less likely to ejaculate because they are told when they are prescribed Revlemid that it corrupts men's semen and causes birth defects. Sex is great, it is the foundation of life on earth, none of us would be here if it weren't for sex. But it is a powerful urge and tends to be misused for base acts of self-sabotage rather than withheld and transmuted for higher purposes. Men recovering should definitely refrain from ejaculation for at least two months and women should likewise do the same, you will feel a tremendous surge of inner energy if you conserve your sexual energy. Sexual thoughts also must be conquered and pushed to the wayside of your mind to experience the full benefit of celibacy, take complete control of your attention and your thoughts. The spiritual power one can gain from celibacy was the original reason why the majority of the religious orders of the world required their priests and leaders to be celibate. Unfortunately, I think the true teachings have been for the most part lost and nowadays it is only a formality not truly understood and practiced by most.

Mental State:

Cultivate in your own mind a powerful and positive mental state. Realize that you don't in fact have "cancer." Reealize that your doctor is just a man or woman like you, and their opinion is just that, an opinion. There isn't some invisible monster living in you known as cancer that you need to fight. All you need to do is supply your body with the materials it needs to build itself up and it will do so. Be careful not to fall in love with the attention you may get from being a "victim" of cancer. Truthfully, a lot of people don't want to fully recover because they have a deep subconscious need for attention and "having cancer" gets people's attention. Don't be lured into this trap, dig deep and toughen up. Use auto suggestion and <u>tell yourself every night before bed "I am getting better every day, in every way"</u> this alone is truly a powerful and profound technique despite being so simple.

Environment:

Our environment has a powerful effect on our mental state. Think about how you feel when you are in a dirty, disorganized place vs. when you are in a clean and organized space. The truth is our environment shapes our mental state in a major way, make sure your environment is clean, organized and exactly how the highest version of yourself demands it to be. The people that occupy our environment and their attitudes are also highly contagious so be sure to keep away any negative people and try and spend your time with positive and upbeat people. Don't allow yourself to be pandered as "the victim." Of course you will be in severe pain if your symptoms are bad and it's OK to be pampered while you are recovering, just don't fall in love with the attention of being the victim.

Attitude is everything:

Our thoughts are real things and they are powerful things. **We become what we think about!** Therefore, take the time to DECIDE who you want to be, and how you want to be remembered and keep working to become that best version of yourself. Realize that your diagnosis is just a speed bump in your journey of life and it will end up making you much stronger after you have conquered it. **THINK RIGHTEOUS THOUGHTS AND YOUR BODY WILL FOLLOW SUIT.**

Reflect Deep:

Do your best to make sure that your subconscious mind and conscious mind are aligned as one. We achieve this by doing things that our true selves want to do. Dig deep and decide if there is anything in your life that you know MUST change, but you have been procrastinating the change or delaying it because you know the change will be painful and or inconvenient. It could be your weight, your marriage, your financial situation, your job or etc. Many times a fresh perspective and cutting through our previously held false beliefs is all we really need, but sometime there are irreparable situations that we know just will never help us reach our goal/ideal and it's better to make the change TODAY. If we don't make a change we will be forever haunted by the situation and it will drain our mental state, if it gets real bad physical symptoms will begin to manifest as a result of the mental anguish as we become what we think about and if we think of pain, frustration and misery we will surely get it eventually.

Chicken Bone Broth Souper Food Recipe:

1) Purchase chicken bones from your local grocery store
2) Add chicken bones to a Stainless Steel Stock Pot (Don't use Aluminum, it leeches into the food!)
3) Add water and a splash of apple cider vinegar to fully cover the chicken bones
4) Add salt (1 Tbsp to start, more to taste at the end)
5) Cook for 8-12 hours on low heat and cool off. A crock pot also works great for this on a low setting
   a. Pour through a sieve to separate the bones and broth (while still hot/warm)
   b. Discard cooked bones
   c. Allow the broth to sit for about an hour and move to the fridge if you aren't using it right away.
   d. The bone broth should turn into a gelatin like texture when it cools down in the refrigerator when cooked properly
6) When ready to make a soup add chicken meat (I use fully cooked rotisserie chicken from supermarket)
7) Add Sliced Carrots, Celery, and onion and cook for about 30-40 minutes until tender
8) Add Dried Thyme for flavor when you add the vegetables
9) Gradually add salt for taste, tasting as you add
10) Voila! You now have one of the most nutritionally satisfying Soups that is amazing for restoring a calcium deficiency.

Medications and Treatments:

I am only comfortable recommending treatments with no adverse side effects and things that I would use myself. Ask your doctor if they can say the same. In all honesty, the person who I know that fully recovered from Multiple Myeloma used both prescribed medications and Calcium, I truly believe that the prescribed medicines were of little value and it was simply the calcium that made them better. Therefore, I don't think the medications will interfere with the calcium supplementation nor do I think the calcium will interfere with most medications prescribed for Myeloma patients, but as always check with your doctor and make your own decisions, question the doctor and always make the final choice yourself as to what you need. I would certainly begin calcium supplementation immediately and see how it makes you feel.

Excerpt from Dr. George W. Carey's *The Biochemic System of Medicine*, 1894

"***CALCAREA PHOSPHORICA.***

Synonym.—*Calcium phosphate.*

Common Name.—*Phosphate of lime. PHOSPHATE OF LIME is destined to play a prominent part in the treatment of the sick, when its range is fully understood by medical practitioners. This salt works with albumen, carries it to bone tissue or to any part of the body where it may be needed. It uses albumen as a cement to build up bone structure.*

Bone is fifty-seven per cent, phosphate of lime, the remainder gelatine; an albuminous, gluey substance, carbonate of soda, magnesium phosphate and sodium chloride. Without the lime phosphate no bone can be made.

When, for any reason, the molecules of this salt fall below the proper standard in the blood, some disturbance in life's processes occur. It may be that bone-cells are not rebuilt as fast as they die. In such cases, if the deficiency exists for a great length of time, a condition of anaemia prevails; for the bone is the basis, the foundation-stone, of the organism. Should the albumen, not having a sufficient quantity of the lime phosphate to properly take care of it, become a disturbing element and be thrown off by the kidney route, the wise (?) men call it Bright's disease. If through the nasal passages, the condition is named catarrh. If by the lungs, a cough is produced. If the albumen reaches the skin, pimples, eruptions, freckles, a condition called eczema, or perchance sores; if the amount at a given point be large, it is sometimes called scrofula. But just what relation the word scrofula has to a running sore is hard to tell, unless it is the fact that the ancients thought those who ate pork were more liable to be thus afflicted. The word is from scrofa—a sow.

Calcium phosphate is found in gastric juice, and a lack of the proper balance is frequently the cause of indigestion. Conditions called rheumatism are sometimes due to a deficiency of the cell-salt. It is well known to Biochemists that a proper balance of sodium phosphate is required to prevent an acid condition from prevailing, and under cer- tain conditions, when calcium phosphate for any reason is not present in proper quantities, the affinities draw upon sodium phosphate in an endeavor to supply the lack, and thus a deficiency in the alkaline salts ensue, which allows an acid condition to prevail, i.e rheumatism.

Calcium phosphate is an auxiliary to the therapeutical effects of magnesium phosphate, as it more nearly resembles that salt than any other. When Magnes. phos. is clearly indicated, and does not restore the normal condition in a reasonable length of time, Calc. phos. should be given, for it is quite certain that it has been drawn on from the blood to assist the work of Magnes. phos., hence the deficiency in the lime-salt.

It is through his understanding of the peculiar workings and affinities of the inorganic salts that the Biochemist is so completely equipped for the battle against so-called disease.

MENTAL SYMPTOMS.—*Peevish, fretful children. Poor memory; incapacity for concentrated thought; mind wanders from one subject to another; weak minds in those practicing, or who have practiced, self-abuse (Kali phos.) . Dull, stupid; depression of spirits; anxious about the future. Desires solitude. After grief, disappointment, pain, etc.*

HEAD.—*Headache, with cold feeling in the head, and head feels cold to the touch. Headache on top of head and behind the ears. Tight sensation. Headache of girls at puberty, with restlessness and nervousness. Headache worse from mental exertion, worse near the sutures. Skull is thin and soft. Closure of the fontanelles delayed or re=opening of same. Vertigo (Ferr. phos.). Crawlings over the head, with cold sensations. Ulcers on top of head.*

Dropsy of the brain, and to prevent these conditions. Loss of hair; bald spots. Inability to hold up the head, owing to a deficiency of lime phospate in the system.

EYES.—*Sensitive to artificial light. Eyeballs ache; spasm of the eyelids (Magnes. phos.). Squinting. Hot feeling in the lids. Paralysis of the retina, causing dimness and loss of sight (Kali phos.). Neuralgic pain in eyes, when Magnes. phos. fails. Inflammation of the eye, with characteristic discharge, especially in scrofulous subjects. Intolerance of light (Ferr. phos.).*

EARS.—*Aching pain, with swelling of the glands of face and neck. Earache, with characteristic albuminous, excoriating discharge. In scrofulous persons, where the glands are much swollen. Ears swollen, burning and itching.*

FACE.—Anaemic, or chlorotic face. Dirty-looking face. Rheumatism of face, which is worse at night. Pimples on the face. Pains in face, with a creeping sensation; feeling of coldness and numbness. Face sallow, pale, earthy; skiri cold and clammy. L,upus. Heat in face. Freckles, eruptions on trie face of young persons, especially of young girls at puberty. Pains in face, of a grinding, tearing nature Magnes. phos.). Pale face in children, when teething is difficult.

MOUTH.—Bad, disgusting taste in mouth in the morning, caused by non-assimilation of food. Consider also Natr* phos.

TEETH.—Retarded dentition (Calc. flnor.). Phosphate of lime is a constituent of the teeth, and when this material is deficient, dentition will be slow and painful, often causing convulsions {Magnes. phos.) and other ailments. Teeth decay as soon as they appear. Gums inflamed and painful (Ferr. phos.). Toothache, which is worse at night (Silicea). Chief remedy in all teething disorders. "If the gums be pale this remedy is especially indicated" (Schuessler).

THROAT.—Enlargement of throat. Goitre (chief remedy) {Natr. mur.). Chronic enlargement of the tonsils. "I have given it in the acute stage, when suffocation threatened, with excellent results " (Chapman). Glands painful, aching; deglutition painful. Thirst, with dry tongue and mouth. Sticking pain in throat on swallowing. Constant hoarseness. Hemming and scraping of throat when talking. Public speakers are greatly benefited by it (alternate with Ferr. phos.). Burning and soreness in larynx and pharynx, in *cases of chronic catarrh, when there is considerable dropping from the posterior nares.*

GASTRIC SYMPTOMS.—*Pain after eating. Food seems to lie in a lump. Heaviness and burning. Pains worse from eating even the smallest amount of food {Ferr. phos.). Stomach sore to the touch. Abnormal appetite, but food causes distress. Cold drinks and food greatly aggravate the pains, while heat relieves (Magnes. phos.). Faint, sinking feelings in region of stomach. Pain sometimes relieved by belching wind. Infants vomit sour, curdled milk {Natr. phos.). Constant desire to nurse. Stomach feels bloated. A course of this remedy should be given after gastric or typhoid fever, and in all cases where digestion is poor, to aid assimilation of food. Vomiting after cold drinks. Headache, accompanied with indigestion. Belching of gas. Most of the gastric symptoms which come under this remedy are due to non-assimilation of food.*

ABDOMEN AND STOOL.—*Diarrhoea in teething children; stools slimy, green undigested, with colic {Natr. phos.) . Give injection of hot water. Cholera infantum, child craves food it should not eat. Stool is hot, often noisy and offensive {Kali phos.). Summer complaint caused from inability to properly digest the food. Diarrhoea after eating green fruit, abdomen sunken. Face pale and anxious, child fretful. Pain in the abdomen near the navel. Infant cries when it nurses. Marasmus, eats heartily but grows more emaciated all the time. Frequent call to stool, but passes nothing {Kali phos., Magnes. phos.). Diarrhoea of school-girls, with the accompanying headache. Costiveness, with hard stool, in old people and infants. Itching piles, also protruding piles {Calc.*

jlitor., Ferr. phos.). Hemorrhoids which ooze an albuminous substance resembling white of egg, especially noticeable in anaemic persons. Cracks and fissures of anus {Calc. finor.). Fistulas without pain. Offensive stools {Kali phos.). Neuralgia of rectum and pain after stool. Symptoms all worse at night or with change of weather {Silicea). To prevent formation of gall-stones.

BACK AND EXTREMTIES.—Calc. phos. being appropriately named "the bone remedy," plays an important part in the symptoms of disease located in the back and extremities, which are largely composed of this material. Curvature of the spine (with mechanical supports}. Numbness and coldness of the limbs. Pains and aching in the joints. Cold sensations in the limbs, as if cold water were being poured over them. Pains in the bones, especially the shin-bones. Pain worse at night and in cold, damp weather. Rheumatism of the joints, and in the back between the shoulders; very severe and worse at night or during rest. Lumbago (Ferr. phos.). Hydroma patella, cysts. Hydrops. Articular spinal irritation. Injuries of the coccyx. Infants are slow in learning to walk, and the bones are soft and friable.

FEBRILE CONDITIONS.—Chilliness and shivering when beginning of fever (Ferr. phos.). Perspiration excessive. Night=sweats in phthisis. Cold, clammy sweat on the face and body. After typhoid and other fevers, as the disease declines, to promote the deposit of new material in place of that destroyed.

MODALITIES.—*Symptoms are generally worse at night in damp, cold weather, and change of weather, getting wet, etc. Better in warm weather and in warm room."*

-The Biochemic System of Medicine, Dr. George W Carey, 1894

Afterword:

I sincerely hope that you found this material helpful, it comes straight from the heart. Please share this with anyone else you know suffering from this dis-ease. A summary is available on my website:

multiplemyeloma-cure.com

Please share the website with anyone else who may be suffering from these symptoms and consider making a donation if you found this information valuable.

Thank You and Stay Strong!

NOTES:

References:

____

[i] https://www.cancer.org/cancer/multiple-myeloma/detection-diagnosis-staging/signs-symptoms.html
[ii] https://d-calusa.com/low-calcium-symptoms-deficiency/